Sunbedyoga

How to exercise and relax on your holiday without leaving your sunbed!

"Just what I needed to help me relax more on my holiday!"..... Brian

Nick Pay

WHAT OTHERS ARE SAYING...

"Required reading for anyone who goes on holiday! An easy way to exercise without feeling I am!"...CeCe (international flight attendant).

"Just what I needed to get me ready for another night of holiday fun!" ....Tim.

Sunbedyoga

How to exercise and relax on your holiday without leaving your sunbed!

Nick Pay

Published in Australia by PL450 Publishing

Postal: P O Box 56, KOOLUNGA, SA, Australia
Email: nicholaspay@hotmail.com
Website: www.tonicbodyandsoul.com

First published in Australia 2013
Copyright © Nick Pay 2013
Cover design, Rogan

Pay, Nick

Sunbedyoga: How to exercise and relax on your holiday
without leaving your sunbed!

ISBN: 978-0-9923620-0-3 PL450 Publishing

8

About the author

Nick worked in and owned a deck-chair hire business by the beach in Adelaide, Australia for almost twenty years. After selling his business and moving to Bali for three years (where he spent a lot of time on sunbeds around pools and by the beach), he returned to Melbourne to study the Advanced Diploma of Yoga Teaching, where he gained the knowledge to finally write this book.

Nick has practised yoga for the last fourteen years, and has now opened a day spa on the beautiful island of Nusa Lembongan where he teaches a relaxation based practice. He is currently in the process of adapting this book for use by the aged and those who are bed-ridden.

He hopes you enjoy this book, and can gain some of the many benefits that occur through the practice of yoga. Most of all he wants you to relax on your holiday!

To Sputnik.

Acknowledgments

I would like to thank everyone who has helped with producing this book, including my illustrator, my editor and my cover designer.

In particular I would like to thank my beautiful, kind, inspiring wife, Josie.

Contents

16

Introduction

Enclosed in this book are practices that will help you feel refreshed and rejuvenated, and to bring greater enjoyment to your holiday. Sometimes when you are on holiday, you know you should exercise but you just don't feel like it! This book has the answer!

Some of the practices are easy to incorporate into your daily life, even when you aren't lucky enough to be holidaying on a sunbed!

Above all, enjoy your holiday and you will be able to return home and tell your friends: "I did lots of yoga on my holiday!"

Brief yoga history

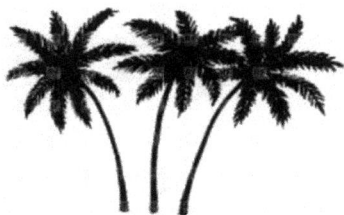

The word yoga comes from Indian Sanskrit and means "to unite". Yoga has existed for over 3000 years, and is a method or practice used to unite the physical body and the mind. These teachings and philosophies take a holistic approach to the individual, focusing on the body, mind, and spirit to create harmony and unity, and to still the fluctuations of the mind.

Around 200 BC the Yoga Sutras of Patanjali were composed. Containing almost two hundred aphorisms on daily life, amongst them is an eight-fold path to enlightenment. It covers instruction on things we should and shouldn't do, physical practices, breath control, control of the senses, increasing the power of concentration, meditation, contemplation and reflection. The sutras also help with guidance of how to overcome barriers to our goal of balance - or unity - within the body and mind. The eight-limb path is not linear and people are often introduced to yoga by the physical postures (or asana).The little bit of quiet time you find when practising asana encourages the investigation of the other limbs or practices.

Yoga was introduced to the West in the late 1800's by travelling Yoga masters who gave demonstrations of yoga postures. There are many different styles of practice and teachings, and there is not one path or the best path, only the path that feels right for you.

Sunbed yoga has been developed through careful consideration of which yoga practices will aid the holidaymaker to undertake some activity to invigorate and nourish the mind and body, with the flow-on effect of increased relaxation and enjoyment while you're away.

Benefits of yoga

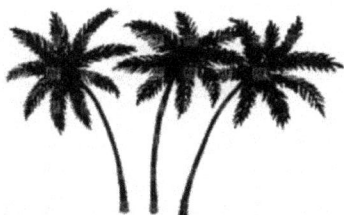

The benefits of yoga have gained a lot of attention over the last few years as westerners have become aware of its benefits. Regular yoga practice is good for the body and the mind as it makes you feel great. The postures are effortless and energise the body rather than tiring it, as the body embraces the positions of yoga practice. Each asana works different parts of the body: both the physical and visible areas, and also the subtle energy levels. The postures not only shape and tone our outside but they work on the inside too. Asana practice is beneficial to the central nervous system, and helps stimulate metabolism and the internal organs. Yoga creates energy and improves stamina, fitness, and concentration as awareness of the body is developed.

It is often said: "it is the mind that starts a yoga practice but it is the body that brings us back!"

Forgetting all the scientific reasons for practising yoga, we do it because it feels GREAT!

How to use this book

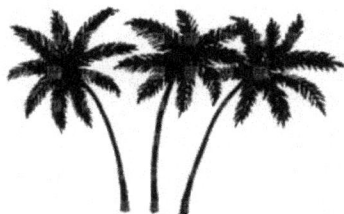

Follow the program as laid out in chapter four of this book. Your breath should be easy during your practice breathing – in and out through your nose. In general, you breathe in as you extend up into a pose, then out as you fold or bring your torso to your knees.

Once the lying and seated postures have been completed you can choose to either finish there or continue to the breathing practice chapter before finishing with the visualisation chapter. There are optional standing poses and some face exercises that can also be performed. To gain the most benefits, the practises should be performed in sequence: lying and sitting postures, standing postures (if you feel up to it), facial exercises and then the visualisation and breathing practice.

The asana sequence is designed to warm up the body without putting extra strain on your muscles. Although you are on holidays, and may eat all day, the exercises are best performed on a relatively empty stomach. If you are concerned about your health or aren't able to complete all of the asana, then do what you can. Stop if anything hurts, if you feel any straining, or just don't feel good about the practice.

Make sure your sunbed is on stable ground.

All the asana should be performed with steadiness and ease – sthiram and stukham – no straining. Your practice should be enjoyable!

Caution should be taken if you are pregnant, have had recent surgeries: heart, spine or joint problems, or high blood pressure. It is always recommended to seek guidance from a doctor before undertaking any new exercise program.

The first rule of yoga practice is to do no harm!

The sunbed yoga practice

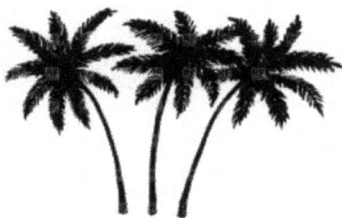

Shavasana or corpse pose

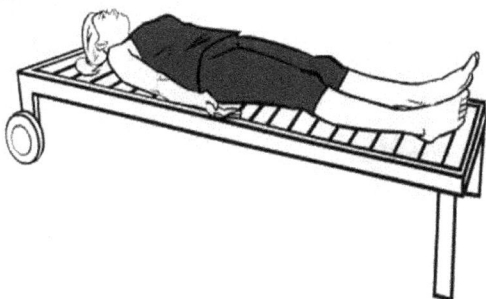

- Relaxes the whole body.
- Calms the nervous system.
- Chance to check in with how you are feeling.

The first asana is 'shavasana' or corpse pose. This is a great way to relax and take stock of your body and how you are feeling in general. It's easy: lie on your back, legs straight and let your feet fall to the sides; lie with your palms facing up. You might like to place a folded towel beneath your head as it is more comfortable if your nose is higher than your chin. Relax and take a few deep, cleansing breaths. This is also the way to lie in the relaxation/visualisation practice.

Ardha (half) Apanasana or wind relieving pose

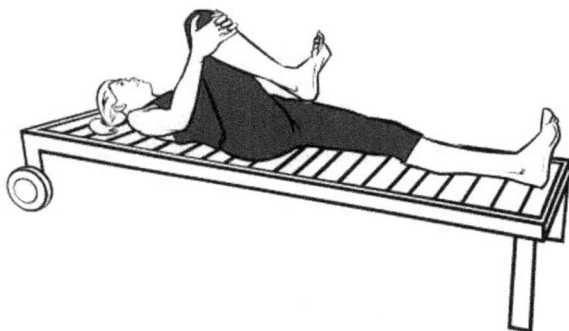

- Massages the stomach.
- Stretches the buttocks.
- Stretches the lower back.

To give your lower back a stretch and massage your stomach, it's as easy as raising your legs! Lift one leg at a time on an inhalation and lower the leg on an out breath. Do this slowly, taking the full length of the breath to raise and lower your leg. When you have raised and lowered each leg three to five times, lift both legs and hold with either your hands on your knees or shins. This will give your belly a really good massage to aid digestion while giving your lower spine a great stretch.

Apanasana or wind relieving pose

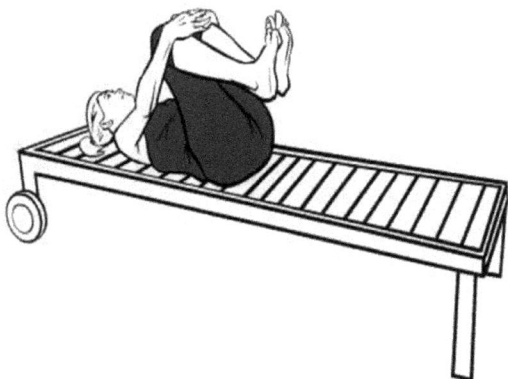

- Lower back stretch.
- Aids digestion.
- Massages internal organs.

Once you have held your legs to your chest for a couple of breaths, try gently rocking back and forward a few times, then try rocking to the left and right. This will give your lower back a really good massage and massage your internal organs. You will also feel your buttocks stretching nicely. After you have completed the rocking, extend both legs straight out and relax in shavasana for a few breaths.

Leg through the hole pose

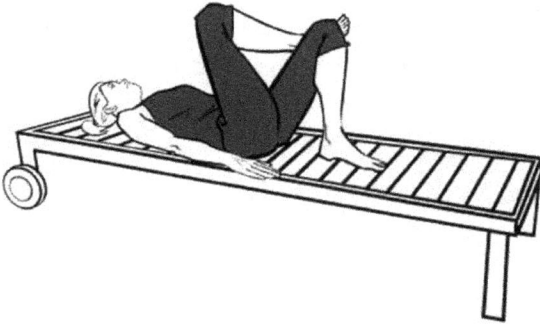

- Stretches the glute muscle.
- Stretches lower back muscles.
- Massages internal organs.

Now place your right foot on your sunbed (a little bit away from your buttocks) and place your left ankle against the bent right knee. Pass your left hand through the hole you have formed and grab your right shin. With your right hand hold the shin of your right leg. You may need to lift the right foot off your sunbed just a little. This should once again give your buttock muscles a good stretch. Hold for a couple of breaths then place your foot back on the sunbed. Do this three times and then repeat with the other leg.

Şetu bandhasana or bridge pose

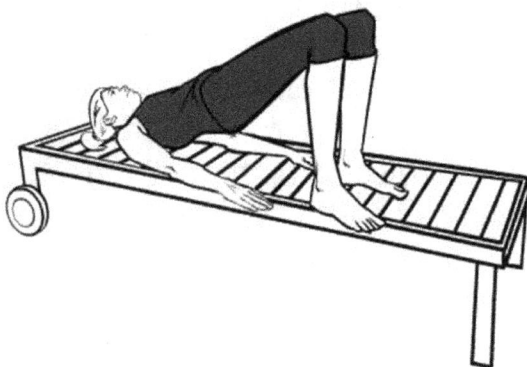

- Opens the chest.
- Strengthens the legs.
- Good for the nervous system.

Bend both your knees and place your feet a short distance away from your buttocks. Keep your arms at the side of the body with the palms facing up. This position is called: 'the constructive rest position', and is great for resting! You

41

can stay like this for a while and then when you are ready, you can move onto the bridge pose.

Breathing in, turn your palms to face down, lift your pelvis off the sunbed a couple of centimetres; hold for a bit then lower on an out-breath. On each in-breath, raise your hips a little higher, lowering as you breathe out. Once again, this is great for the lower back and your abdomen. It also helps to stretch the front of your body and is a slight inversion increasing the blood flow to the brain. Do three to five of these bridge poses, and then once you're finished, bring both knees into your chest before transitioning into the constructive rest position. Be very careful if you have any issues with your neck!

Vipariti karani or raised legs

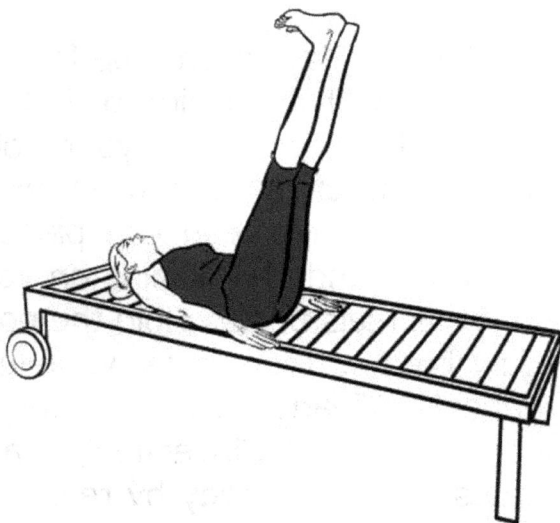

- Improves lower body circulation.
- Relaxes the nervous system.
- Great after a day walking or a night dancing!

Lying on your back in shavasana with your arms at your sides, bring your knees to your chest and then straighten your legs. If you have tight hamstrings, you may have difficulty straightening your legs completely. Be careful if you have hip problems.

Vipariti karani is often performed against a wall with a cushion or bolster under your hips. Try this in your hotel room at the end of the day for an extra relaxation experience. You can place a rolled-up towel under your hips on your sunbed if this feels better. Hold the pose for a few breaths then lower your legs and repeat. Vipariti karani pose is classified as an 'inversion', and invigorates the whole body by reversing the effects of gravity.

Easy side twist

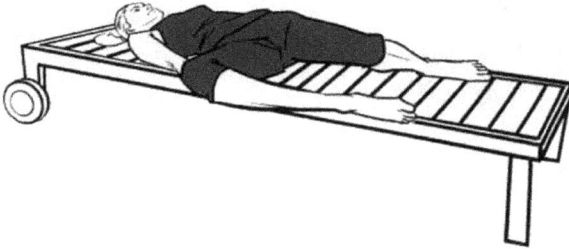

- Stimulates and tones internal organs.
- Good for the waistline.
- Good for digestion.

Lying on your back with your upper torso relaxed, bend your knees and place your feet on the outside edges of your sunbed. On an out-breath, lower your knees to one side feeling the luxurious stretch across the lower back and stay in this position for a few breaths. On an in-breath, return your knees to the upright position then lower to the opposite side on an out breath. Repeat three to five times. Relax once again in shavasana, and then when you are ready raise yourself into a sitting position.

Dandasana or staff pose

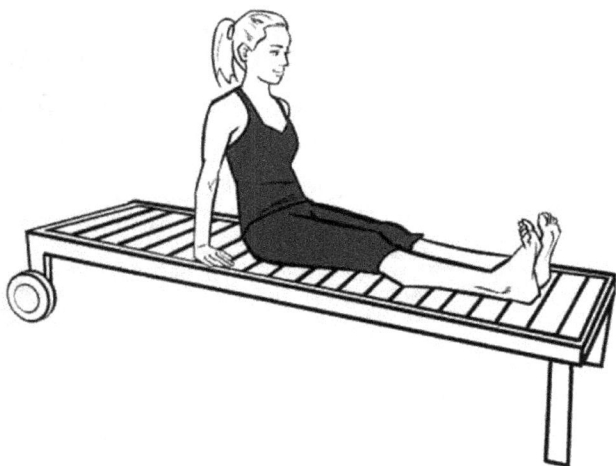

- Opens the front of the chest.
- Great for body awareness.
- Brings consciousness to your posture.

Time to sit up now; do it slowly if you have been lying for a while! Sit with your legs straight out in front of you, arms relaxed at your sides. Breathe in and straighten your spine from your coccyx to the base of the skull. Breathe out, retaining your stretched spine, and relax your shoulders. Relax your jaw and lower your chin, slightly stretching the back of your neck, looking forward and breathe normally. This is great for the posture, leg muscles, and can bring an awareness of the body.

Navasana or boat pose

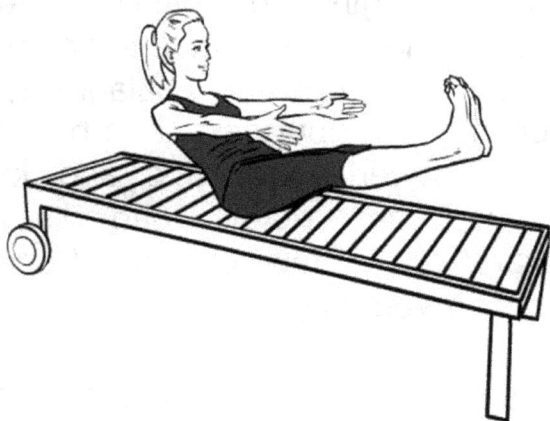

- Really stimulates the abdomen, helping with gastric problems.
- Great for the waistline.
- Strengthens the back.

Navasana is the most strenuous pose of the program, and can be left out if you feel you are not up to it. Sit in the staff pose, with your spine nice and straight then lean your body backwards to an angle of about 60 degrees. Then raise your feet – legs straight, if you can. Next, raise your arms directly in front of you, keeping them straight at shoulder level and bringing the palms to the outside of the knees, fingers pointing forward. Hold the posture, balancing on the bones of your buttocks, and breathe normally. Lower your arms and legs when you are ready, and lie in shavasana for a few breaths. Repeat five times if you have the energy.

Remember to keep the spine straight; this will give you a nice stretch across your chest. Be careful if you have high blood pressure.
An easier version of this pose is to keep your legs bent and your hands by your sides.

Sun breaths

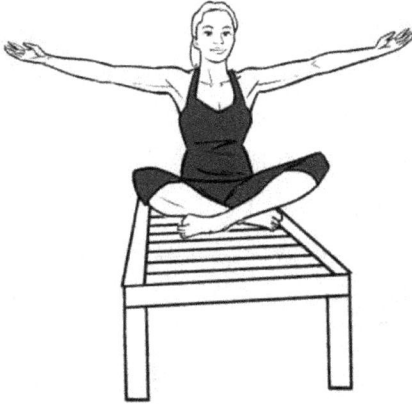

- Invigorates the whole body with fresh air.
- Increases circulation.
- Relaxes the nervous system.

Sun breaths can be performed seated, or you can also complete them at the end of the sunbed practice in the standing section.

Sit in an easy position with your legs crossed, or if you prefer, you can do sun breaths in a kneeling or standing position. It may be more comfortable if you place a rolled up towel beneath your buttocks if you are seated. As you inhale raise your arms above your head, looking up as you do so. As you breathe out, lower your arms. Take the time of the full breath to raise and lower your arms. Feel how invigorating this is as your body becomes flushed with fresh oxygen. Do this ten times. It is nice to then sit with your eyes closed and experience the effects of this wonderful asana.

Baddha konasana or cobbler pose

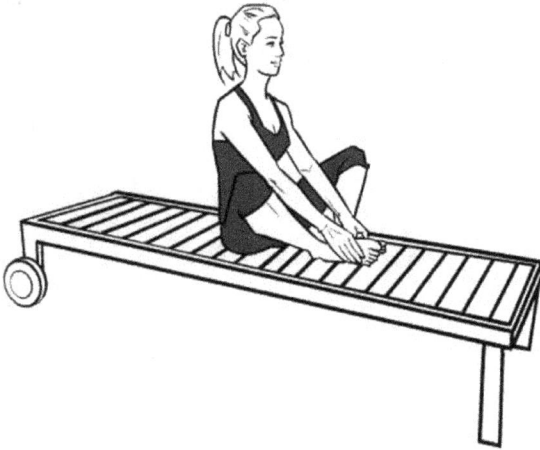

- Stretches leg muscles.
- Good for the lower back.
- Stretches the groin.

The next pose stimulates the abdominals, providing a nice stretch for the groin. Sitting up again, spine nice and straight, breathe in and bend your knees, bringing the soles of your feet together. Allow your knees to fall gently to the sides. You can either hold your feet, or rest your hands lightly on your knees. Take five breaths, then on an in-breath use your hands to bring your knees together, then straighten your legs. Now for a forward bend!

Paschimottanasana or seated forward bend

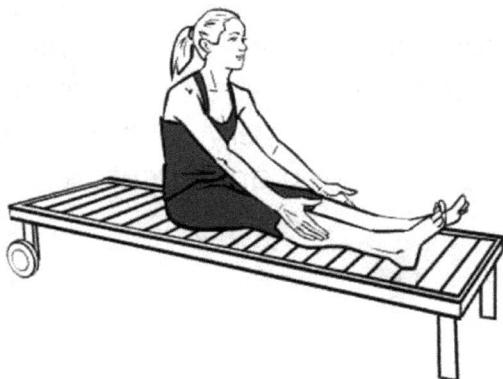

- Stretches the back of the body.
- Improves digestion and circulation.
- Massages the internal organs.

Once again, sit in dandasana, breathe in and pivot forward, bending at the hips. Place your hands anywhere you are comfortable. Keep your back straight, lengthening the spine from the coccyx to the base of the skull. On an exhale, keeping the spine extended, try and lower your chest to your thighs. Be careful not to push too far. Hold for a couple breaths relaxing the muscles while stretching the back of the body. It is important to bend from the hips. And keep the back straight when first bending. This is very calming, and is great for digestion and circulation.

Bharadvajasana or simple twist

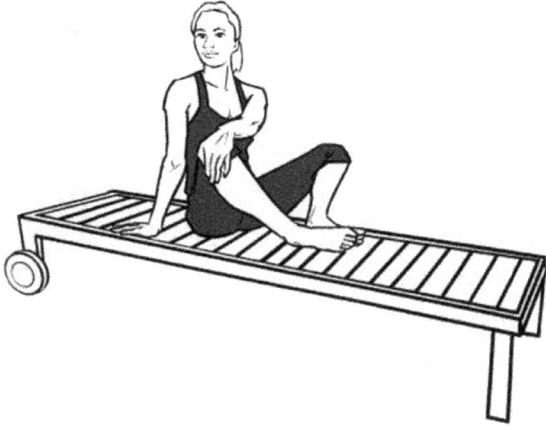

- Strengthens and re-aligns the spine.
- Massages the internal organs.
- Aids digestion.

Starting to twist the spine now. This should be done very carefully, and you should engage an easy twist to begin with. You can sit with your legs crossed, kneel, or choose the badha konasana pose. Place your left hand on your right knee and breathe in deeply. Breathing out, twist gently to your right. Make sure you keep your spine upright and look over your right shoulder if you don't have neck issues. Breathing in, make sure your spine is erect, and then on the next exhale twist that little bit more. Do this a couple more times while maintaining your breathing, and when you are ready, on an in-breath face toward the front. Repeat on the other side: right hand on left knee and look over your left shoulder.

Cow and cat pose

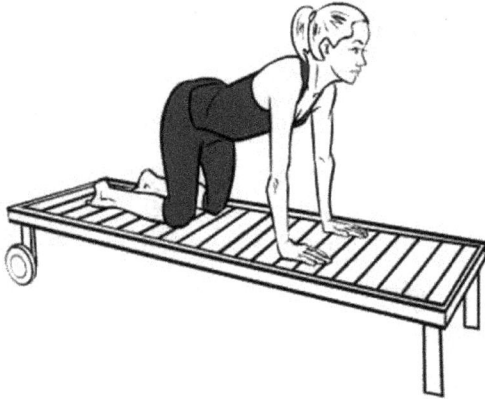

- Improves circulation and digestion.
- Flexes the spine.
- Strengthens the arms and backs.

Time to move to your hands and knees. Be careful if you have sore wrists or issues with your knees or back.

Once again, make sure your sunbed is nice and stable.

These poses are called the cat to cow sequence. In this sequence, the hands and knees remain stationary and you only want to move your spine. With straight arms, place your hands under your shoulders and your knees directly in line with your hips. Exhale as you round your back, bringing your chin to your chest (this is the cat part). Then inhale, looking up as you gently dip your spine (the cow part). Using a slow, full breath, repeat the process, imagining you are a cat arching its spine in the sun – giving you a nice stretch at the same time.

Urdhva hastasana

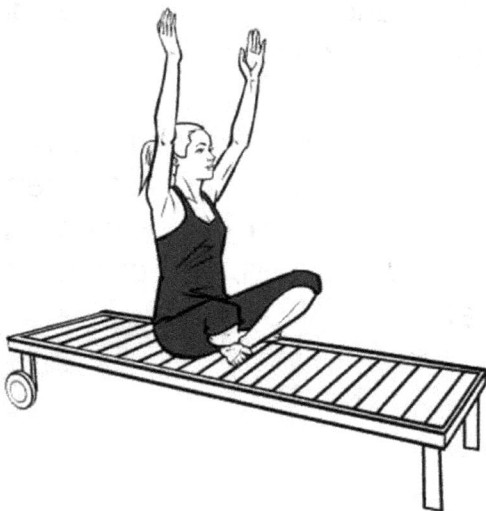

- Stretches the sides.
- Elongates the spine.
- Stimulates the internal organs.

Raising your arms above your head stretches the sides of the body and helps to elongate the spine. This asana can be practised either seated on your sunbed or later in the standing section. With your arms raised, gently lean over to one side on an out-breath and then return to neutral on an in-breath. Then repeat on the other side. You don't need to bend very much to gain a wonderful side-stretch.

Remember to bend the same amount of times on both sides, and to keep your spine upright during the practice. If you have shoulder issues, you can keep your hands at your sides.

Childs pose or balasana

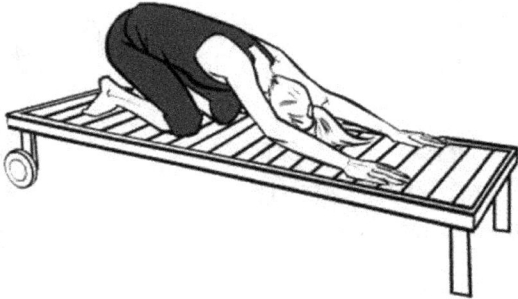

- Relaxes the body.
- Stretches the spine.
- Increases blood flow to the face.

Time for a bit of a rest.

From your hands and knees, lower your bottom to your heels and bring your forehead to the sunbed. This must be done carefully for those with knee problems. If your head doesn't reach the sunbed, you can form two fists and rest your forehead on them. You can either place your arms along the sides of your legs or out in front of you. Remember, this is a relaxation asana, you should feel relaxed!

Rest here for as long as you like while maintaining steady, natural breathing.

For those of you with blood pressure issues, be careful when you sit up. Enjoy and explore the relaxing feeling of this great pose.

Cobra pose

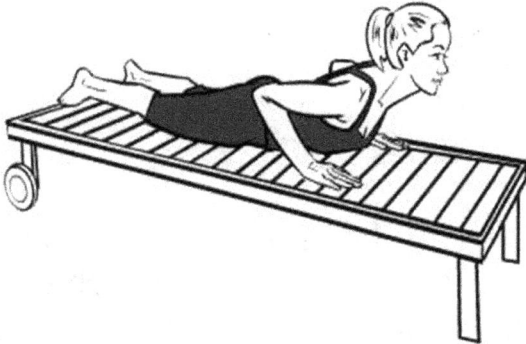

- Strengthens the chest.
- Massages abdominals.
- Strengthens the lower back.

Moving forward from your kneeling position, lie on your stomach with your hands flat on the sunbed, level with your chest. Breathing in, move your hands forward to bring your elbows under the line of your shoulders, raising your chest off the sunbed. Breathe evenly, and after three of four breaths, lower on an exhale. Repeat a couple of times.

Another option here is to extend the arms in front of you and lift the arms and legs at the same time on an in breathe and then relax again on your sunbed on an out breath. Repeat three to five times.

After you have completed the cobra pose, you can lie on your stomach for a moment or two, and then roll onto your back into shavasana.

You now have a choice (I know it can be hard making decisions on your holiday); you can continue on to the breathing and relaxation practices, or perhaps you are feeling energised and wish to perform the standing poses.

The Breathing practice

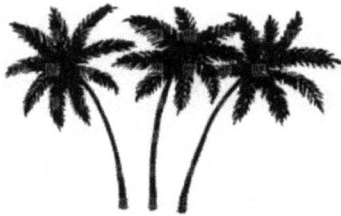

In Patanjali's yoga sutras and his eight-fold path to enlightenment, he names Pranayama, or breath control, as the fourth limb. Prana has different meanings; it can mean breath, life force and energy. Yama means discipline. Breath control leads to control of the mind, which is necessary for concentration and meditation. When we breathe, we stimulate our inner energy (prana, or life force). The use of breath-control during yoga practice is what separates yoga from regular physical exercise.

In our daily lives we rarely use the full capacity of our lungs; often only using the top third of our lungs.
In yoga the breath is used to direct the flow of prana, or life force, in the body. Like blood flows through the body along a series of arteries and veins, life force is said to flow along a series or network of pathways called 'nadis' of which there are over 72,000! These nadis meet throughout the body at energy centres called 'chakras'. There are seven major

chakras running along the spine, and these chakras can become blocked. Regular asana practice and Pranayama (breathing practice) can help unblock the chakras.

Pranayama can be a very strong practice, and care should be taken. If you start to feel dizzy, or your breathing becomes erratic, you should stop immediately and lie down, returning to your natural breathing. You may even become over-emotional, in which case, you should stop the practice. If you find you wish to take your Pranayama further, as with all yoga practices there is no substitute for a qualified teacher.

The following practices are included here to introduce you to three simple techniques to improve your breath.

The first practice is called the 'full yogic breath'. It can be useful to place the hands on the belly to gain awareness of what is happening when you breathe. As you breathe in, try and breathe to the lower part of your lungs. You may feel a sensation of your belly rising. This provides a massage of the internal organs. As you continue to breathe in, try to feel the sides of the rib cage expanding. For the final part of the practice, try and feel the breath expanding across your upper torso and shoulder region. You can release the breath by relaxing the abdomen region first, then the sides, and finally the upper torso area. Continue this for a few minutes. Over time this method of breathing will increase the lung capacity, and the effect of deep breathing will invigorate the whole body.

The second method of breathing will help calm the body and mind. It is called 'nadi sodana' or 'alternate nostril breathing'. Take your right hand and place your index and middle fingers on your forehead just above the brow. Block off your right nostril with the thumb and breathe in slowly and fully through your left nostril. Then block your left nostril with the little finger and breathe out slowly and steadily through your right nostril. Pause, and then inhale through your right nostril, breathing out through your left nostril. This completes one round. Repeat this for three rounds then return to normal breathing. You can increase the number of rounds after practicing for a while.

The next breath is a little easier. Poke your tongue out and roll it into a tube. Breathe in slowly and deeply through your mouth. Bring your tongue in then close your mouth, breathing out slowly through your nose. Repeat this a few times. This is a cooling and relaxing breath.

The relaxation practice

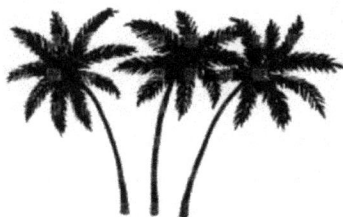

Congratulations on completing your first session of sunbed yoga! If you came to this section first – welcome!

In this chapter I will provide you with visualisation and relaxation techniques to help you unwind on your holiday, but this is also something you can take home with you.

The idea is to place a vivid picture in your mind of your surroundings and the sensations you are feeling while on holiday. This enables you to use this visualisation when you return to the hustle and bustle of your regular life. Maybe there is someone with you who can read this visualisation to you, or perhaps you could record these words on your phone to play back to yourself.

Starting now, you can either sit upright at the end of your sun bed placing your feet on the ground, or you can lie down in shavasana – whichever is the most comfortable for you. Once you feel you are comfortable, take another couple of minutes to make yourself that little bit more comfortable. Maybe you could move your feet further apart or wriggle the whole body just once more. This visualisation will take about ten minutes, and you will feel completely relaxed and, hopefully, completely calm.

Start by looking around you. Notice everything: the clouds and nearby water, the pool, the ocean, palm trees, the   people.   Everything.   Notice everything. Even the tiniest detail of your surroundings will increase the richness of your visualisation. This should put a smile on your face. Be consciously aware of your surroundings and the sensations you are feeling.

Now close your eyes and relax. Give yourself permission to take this time to really relax and forget about anything that worries you, be it in your home-life, work-life, or any other worries you may have. While you are on holiday, these worries do not matter in this moment. During this visualisation, other thoughts may enter your mind. Acknowledge them and put them aside for further consideration. They do not concern you at this point in time. Just breathe in and out, your natural breath, in and out.

Now take three full, deep breaths. With each exhale feel a sense of release, relief and of letting go. Feel your body relaxing. Feel your sunbed beneath you – strong, solid, and unmoving. Focus on the breathe moving into the body and the air moving out of the body.

Allow your body to relax into your position. Feel your face becoming soft, feel your whole body becoming soft, relaxed, and calm.

Now leave the breath for a moment and focus on the sounds around you. Listen to one sound; focus all your attention on that sound. Really listen to it. Enjoy that sound as a sound of your holiday. Now find another sound and concentrate on it. Then find another, and another, always focusing on the current sound and discovering what it is before moving on to the next sound and leaving a picture imprinted in your mind of what is causing that sound. Start to focus on sounds closer to you: the sound of your own breath, in and out, experiencing the gift of life we all share.

Now visualising your surroundings, still with your eyes closed, remember everything you could see: the pool, palm trees, the reflection of the sun on the cool pool water. Remember this picture of your holiday – a calm time, a place of relaxation. Notice everything. Remember everything.

Now feel the warmth of the sun on your body, perhaps the joy of a slight breeze on your skin. Really feel it. Feel it on your toes, your legs, your arms, your torso, and your head. Feel the warmth from the sun, and the coolness and joy of the breeze on your skin. Really feel it, and remember it.

Leave the body for a moment and imagine it in the surroundings you have pictured. Visualise your body in those surroundings – warm, happy, relaxed.

Now leave those thoughts and memories, and come back to your physical body. Feel your sunbed beneath you, still, solid and unmoving. Remember where you are, what time it is, and what you have been doing. Thank yourself for giving you your holiday and this special time to relax. Start to focus on your breath again, feeling your relaxed body. Focus on the breath coming in and out of your nose; your chest expanding and relaxing. Remember the memories you have created – you can take them with you wherever you are.

You may want to rub your hands together to create some warmth then cup your palms over your eyes. Now open your eyes and blink a couple of times. Remove your hands when you are completely ready to rejoin the world, rejoin the place where you are on holiday.

I hope you enjoyed this visualisation; it really is something you can take home with you to your regular life. If you are feeling stressed or need a break, close your eyes and imagine you are on your sunbed by the pool. Remember and re-live the memories and sensations that you have created and enjoy them, again and again.

Standing poses option

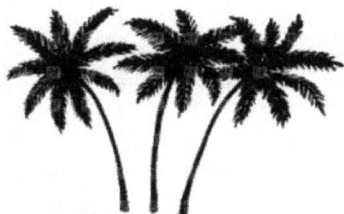

After completing the sunbed yoga section of this book, you may want to perform a handful of standing asana. Be careful when you stand after being seated or lying – you want to give the blood time to return to your head.

Standing poses can strengthen the feet, leg muscles, shoulders, arms, the torso, and pelvis. Standing poses help stimulate blood flow, and can provide a sense of stability and grounding.

Once again remember to practice all asana with steadiness and ease. Nothing should hurt or feel that you are straining.

Your posture and body-alignment in standing poses can give an insight into areas of weakness that can be improved through the practice of yoga.

Tadasana or mountain pose

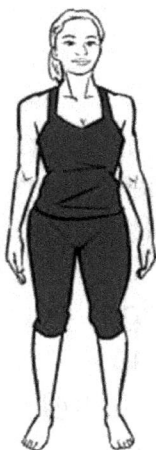

- Provides a sense of grounding.
- Helps your posture.
- Calming.

The first standing asana is 'tadasana' or 'mountain pose'. Tadasana is the basis for all other standing poses.

Stand with your feet either together or a little way apart, and distribute your weight evenly over your feet. Draw up the arches of your feet and relax the muscles around the knees. Arms and hands should be relaxed at your sides. Release and relax your shoulders, then relax and slightly lower your chin. You should feel as if there is an invisible string pulling the crown of your head to the sky. Finally look forward and smile!

Maintain an upright posture and breathe normally. You can close your eyes if you feel comfortable doing so.

Virabhadrasana or warrior pose

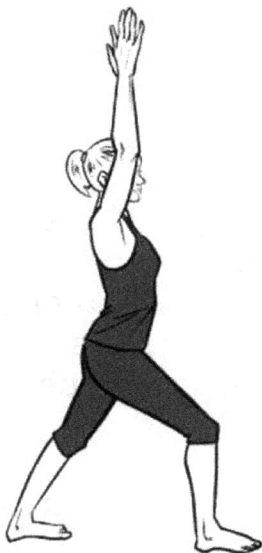

- strengthens the legs, ankles, and knees.
- increases stamina.
- good for overall mental being.

Standing in tadasana, take a step forward with your right leg. Bend your right knee until it is directly above the ankle (you should be able to see your toes over the top of your knee). Turn your left foot slightly outwards, which will help align your body and square off your hips with your front foot. Looking forward, push down through your feet, and breathing in, raise your hands to the sky.

Feel the strength of the warrior within this pose. Hold for a minute, breathing steadily and easily. Lower your arms on an out-breath then stepping forward return to tadasana. Repeat with the left foot forward.

Vrksasana or tree pose

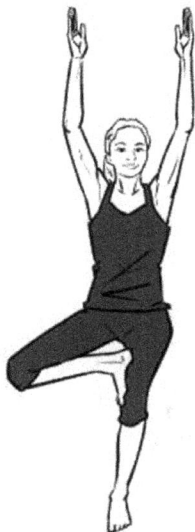

- aids concentration
- good for posture
- improves balance and co-ordination

Once again, stand in mountain pose, keeping your right leg straight and strong. Bend your left leg and place the sole of your foot anywhere on the right leg – except on the knee! The higher you place your left foot the better, right up to the groin if you can. It is also okay to simply put your left foot on your right foot and balance that way. You will still gain the benefits of balance in this pose.

When you are steady, breathe in and raise your arms above your head, forming the branches of the tree. After a few breaths, lower your arms on an exhale, coming out of the pose slowly. Repeat on the other side, and then return to tadasana.

Utkatasana or standing squat

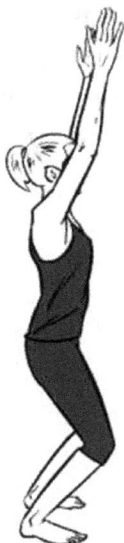

- energises the legs.
- focuses the mind.
- strengthens the feet .

Standing in tadasana, breathe in and raise your arms above your head with your palms facing each other. As you exhale, bend your knees, and if you are up to it on your holiday, lower your torso until your thigh bones are parallel to the ground. It is perfectly okay to lower your torso just a little and hold for a few breaths, then return to tadasana on an in-breathe. This is quite a tiring asana, take it easy, especially if you have sore knees.

Uttanasana or standing forward bend.

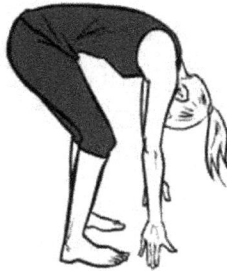

- great for upper body circulation.
- calms and energises the body.
- relaxes neck and shoulder muscles.

Forward bends tend to have a cooling and calming effect on the body and mind. Exhalation during forward bends massages internal organs, and the compression on the pelvic area increases circulation, which has a cleansing effect and brings vitality to the body.

Standing in tadasana, raise your arms above your head and on an out-breath bend forward from your hips, bringing the torso toward the legs. If your hamstrings are tight, or you have lower back issues, it is okay to bend your legs. Breathe easily and steadily, and when you are ready, return to tadasana. Be careful as you stand if you have high or low blood pressure.

You have now completed the standing portion of this practice and you can return to your sunbed and lie in shavasana and relax ready for the visualisation.

Something for the face

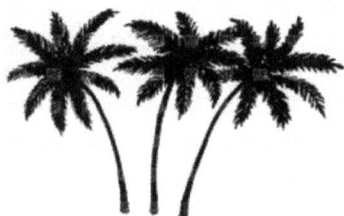

General yoga practice is great for the skin and complexion due to its invigorating and nourishing effects on the whole body.

Facial muscles are no different to other muscles of the body. If you want them to remain firm, they need to be exercised. Perhaps you can practice in front of the mirror.

Try the following three exercises for your face. You can practice on the comfort of your sun bed or in front of a mirror.

You could even practice these exercises when you return home, or even if you get stuck in traffic on the way to and from work! Really, these three exercises can be performed anywhere!

With constant practice you may see a reduction in lines, wrinkles, and bags under your eyes, and you can return from your holiday looking more youthful and invigorated!

Sitting upright on your sunbed in dandasana, think happy thoughts and smile! It is easy you are on holiday! As you smile, release any tension as you smile the biggest smile you can. Bare those teeth and make it big, it won't hurt you! Relax and then smile again. Look around your surroundings and find someone to smile at, you are doing both of you a favour and energising your facial muscles at the same time. Smiling uses a lot of facial muscles and makes you feel good.

The second facial exercise involves blowing the cheeks full of air then circulating the air around the mouth. Fill up your mouth with air and swish it around until you are out of breath. Take another breath and repeat this action three of four times. This provides a good internal massage of the cheeks and stretches and promotes blood flow.

Tilt your head back and try and kiss the ceiling. That's right, pucker up and try and kiss the ceiling! Feel the stretch at the front of your neck as you try to kiss the ceiling. This is great for flushing the lips with blood, and for those tiny lines that appear around the mouth.

Remember there are lots of muscles in the face and they all need exercise to keep them firm. Smiling is a great way to work them!

In conclusion

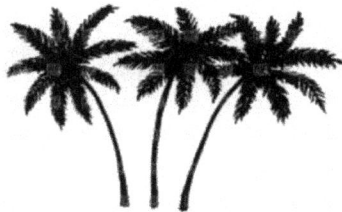

I hope you have enjoyed the sunbed yoga book. Contained within are practices that will stimulate and invigorate the body and mind, improve digestion and help you sleep better, helping you to have a more relaxing holiday.

I hope you enjoy your holiday and your new found yoga practice. Just remember to make sure your sunbed is on stable ground and that if something hurts, DON'T DO IT!

Remember to take things slowly, breathe and do plenty of exercise without leaving your sunbed!

index

References and extra reading

Light on Yoga, B.K.S. Iyengar, (Thorsons 2001)

Asana Pranayama Mudra Bandha, Swami Satyananda Saraswati (Yoga Education Trust)

The Bhagavad Gita, (Faber and Faber)

Useful Contacts

To find Qualified teachers and classes go to:

www.yogaaustralia.org

Want to organise a retreat to practice sunbed yoga?

www.tonicbodyandsoul.com

To order a copy of this book, please go to

www.tonicbodyandsoul.com

or

www.amazon.com

**How did you find this book? Nick would love to hear your feedback or your own story.
Please email your name and comments to nicholaspay@hotmail.com**

notes

notes

notes

www.ingramcontent.com/pod-product-compliance
Lightning Source LLC
Chambersburg PA
CBHW050535280326
41933CB00011B/1593